Stretching

Simple Exercises to Make You Limber

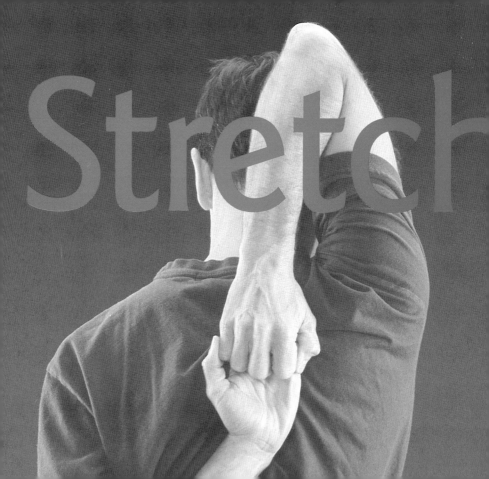

ing

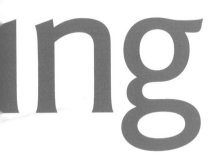
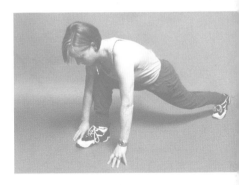

Simple Exercises to Make You Limber

Manine Rosa Golden with Mark Hofer
Photographs by Robert Vinnedge

Andrews and McMeel
A Universal Press Syndicate Company
Kansas City

Designed by Ed Marquand with assistance by Jesianne Asagi

Printed by Midas Printing Limited

Library of Congress Cataloging-in-Publication Data

Golden, Manine Rosa, 1969–
    Stretching : simple exercises to make you limber / Manine Rosa Golden, with Mark Hofer ; photographs by Robert Vinnedge.
        p.   cm.
    ISBN 0-8362-2892-8 (pbk.)
    1. Stretching exercises.   I. Hofer, Mark.   II. Title.
RA781.63.G65   1997
613.7'1—dc21   96-48017
                                                                         CIP

Contents

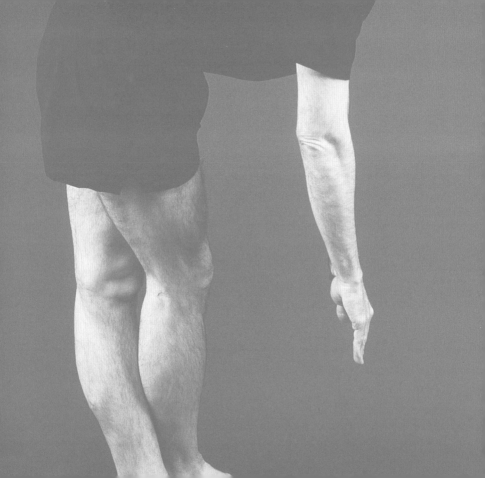

Introduction

Stretching is one of the most important acts you can perform for better health, yet it is often the most neglected part of a person's regular health regime. Stretching should be the first sport that active people learn, but it is often the last. Whether you're a professional athlete or you haven't exercised in years, odds are you don't stretch enough. Regular stretching is the first step to enjoyable, low-stress fitness.

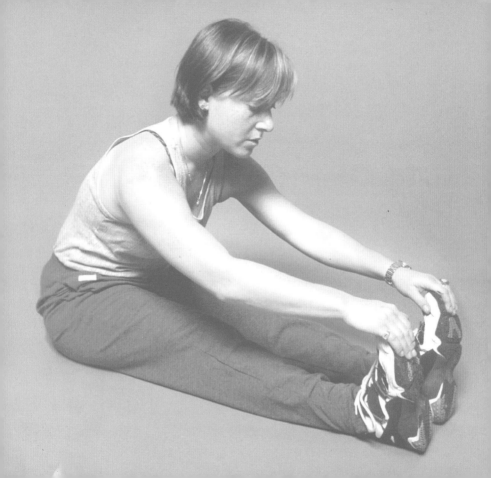

Stretching will show you in minutes
how to improve your health and fitness,
reduce your risk of injury, and become
more limber regardless of your age or
physical condition. Follow the simple pro-
gram illustrated in this book to warm up
your body before more strenuous exercise,
or use the stretches as exercises in them-
selves. Either way, by increasing your range
of motion, strength, coordination, and
flexibility, you will improve your circula-
tion, muscle tone, posture, and self-image.

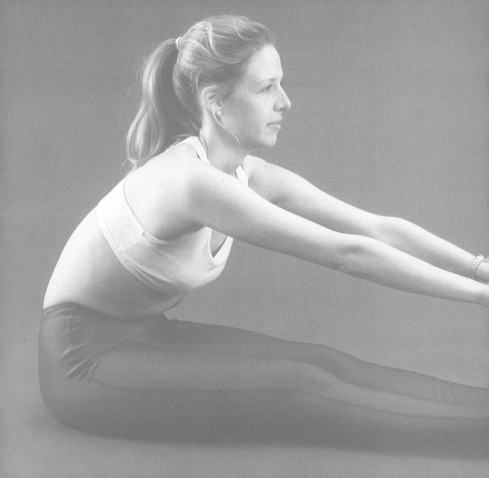

This book illustrates the most basic stretches for each of the major muscle groups in your body and tells you how to get the most out of each stretch. It will teach you a simple, relaxing, and injury-free approach to fitness.

Stretching is an important transition between inactivity and strenuous activity, and should be done both before and after exercise. It is also an effective reliever of stress and an energizer to combat stiffness or sluggishness. Regular stretching reduces muscle tension and promotes freer movement. Stretching should be comfortable and relaxing. Never stretch to the point of pain. Remember, stretching is not competitive. You should work at your own pace and within your own range of comfort, stamina, and flexibility. If you do experience discomfort in the most basic stretches, you should consult your doctor.

How to Stretch

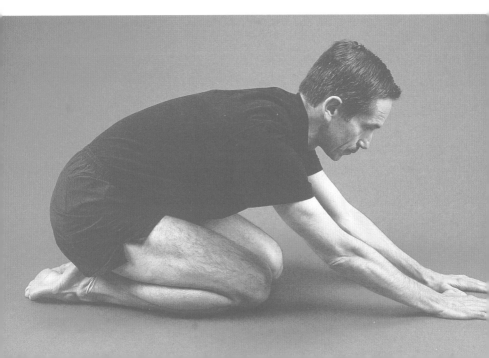

Effectively

Stretching should be treated as a sport and given the same attention as any other sport in which you participate. Before you begin your stretches, you must warm up to get blood to your muscles and loosen your joints. Ten minutes of brisk walking or riding a stationary bike should prepare you for stretching. Before you decide when to fit stretching into your schedule, consider the fact that your body temperature peaks during the middle of the day, and is lowest early in the morning. If you decide to stretch in the morning, it may take your body longer to warm up than if you stretch after work. Listen to what your body tells you. Wear loose clothing and stretch in a room of a comfortable temperature.

When you execute your stretches, never bounce. When muscle fibers are stretched too far, the protective "stretch reflex" in the tissue sends a signal to the brain to contract the muscle. This keeps the tissue from tearing. Therefore, if you stretch too far, you're actually contracting muscles instead of stretching them. Pushing a stretch too far or

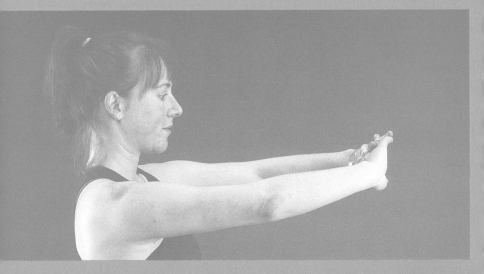

bouncing up and down stimulates the stretch reflex. Always remember to breathe deeply and regularly while you stretch. Exhale as you bend into a stretch and breathe in a controlled, rhythmic manner while you are in the stretch. *A stretch should never be painful.* It should be a lengthening that works with your body, not against it.

Begin each stretch by following the instructions to the point of light tightness and hold that position for 15 to 30 seconds. Relax. Go into the stretch again, this time slightly farther, and hold the stretch for another 15 to 30 seconds. Now go on to the next stretch. If you notice particular tightness in an area, spend more time there than usual. Take each stretch slowly, concentrating on the part of your body and the muscles that you are attending to. Remember that it is not the number of seconds you spend in a stretch that makes it effective, but the amount of focus and attention you give to that part of your body.

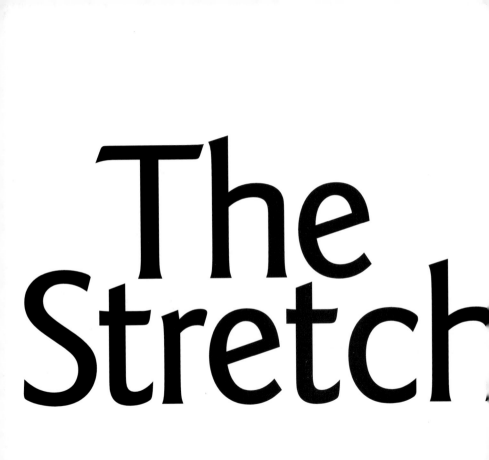

The
Stretch

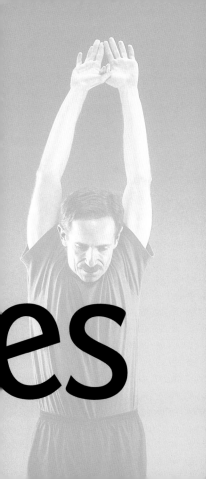

es

Following are stretches for each of the major parts of the body. You may not need to perform all of the stretches all of the time. Try them all first, and then decide which will prepare you best for the activity you are about to perform. You'll find that the stretches you need before and after typing at a desk are different than those you need before and after running.

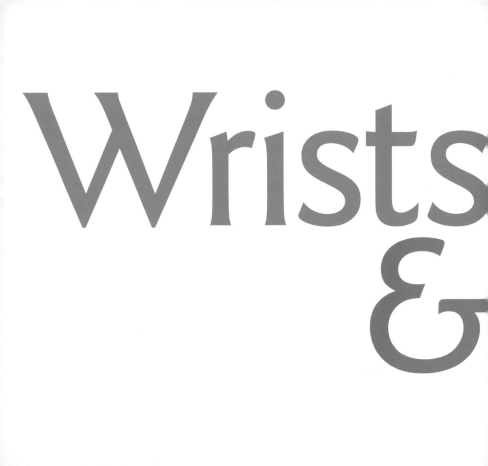

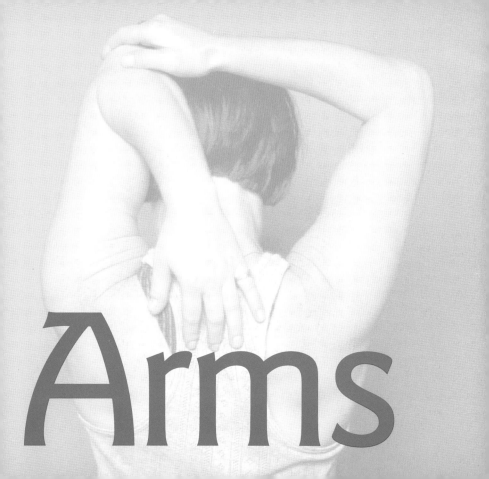

Arms

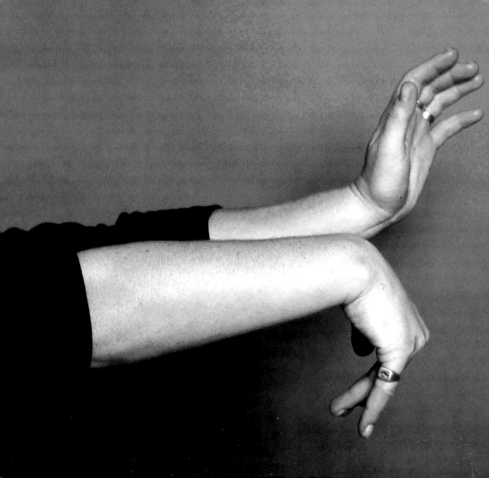

*a simple activity to
prepare joints used
throughout the day in
a variety of activities*

Wrists

Sitting or standing, reach your arms out in front of
you and rotate each of your wrists 10 times in a row
in a clockwise direction and 10 times in a row in a
counterclockwise direction.

You can do a similar stretch for your ankles. Sitting in
a chair or on the floor, rotate each ankle 10 times in
a clockwise direction and 10 times in a counterclockwise direction.

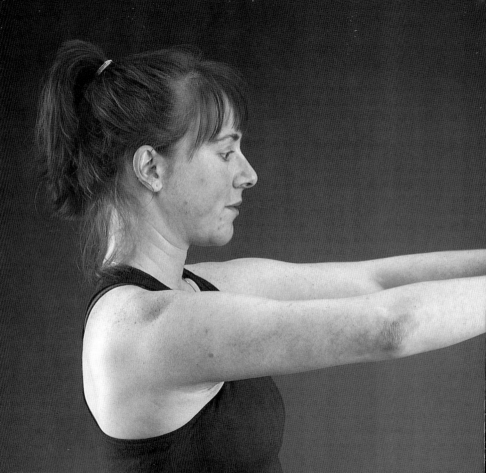

Arms & Hands

Sitting or standing, interlace your fingers in front of your chest at shoulder height. Turn your palms away from your body and extend your arms forward until you feel a stretch in your upper back, shoulders, arms, and hands. Hold this stretch for at least 15 seconds, relax, then repeat it. Next, interlace your fingers above your head. With your palms facing the ceiling, stretch your arms up and slightly back. Hold the stretch for at least 15 seconds, relax, and repeat the stretch for another 15 to 30 seconds.

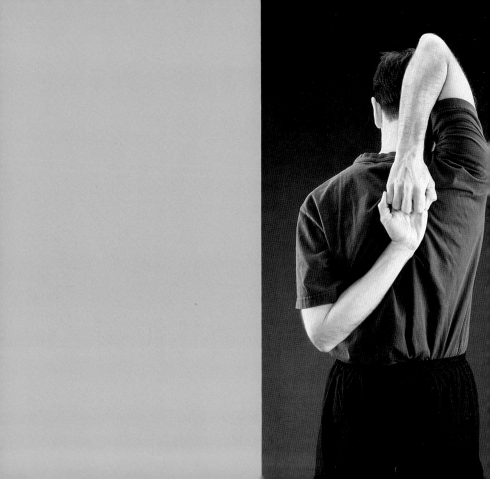

Triceps

Sitting or standing, reach your right arm back over your shoulder and try to touch your right shoulder blade with your right hand. If you can, reach your left hand behind your back, under your shoulder, and try to interlace your right and left hands. Hold the stretch for at least 15 seconds, relax, and repeat the stretch for another 15 to 30 seconds. Relax both arms in front of you, then repeat the stretch on your left arm.

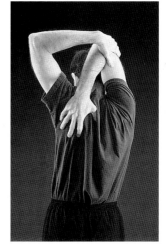

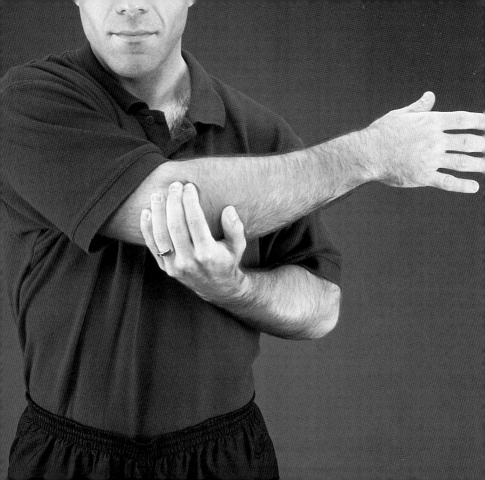

a great stretch to lengthen muscles between the shoulder blades

Arms & Shoulders

Sitting or standing, lift your right arm out in front of you and across your chest. With your left hand on your right elbow, pull your right arm into your chest. Hold the stretch for at least 15 seconds, relax, and repeat it for another 15 to 30 seconds. Repeat the stretch on your left arm.

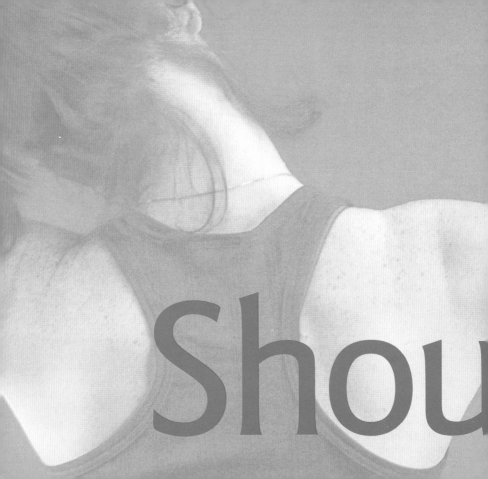

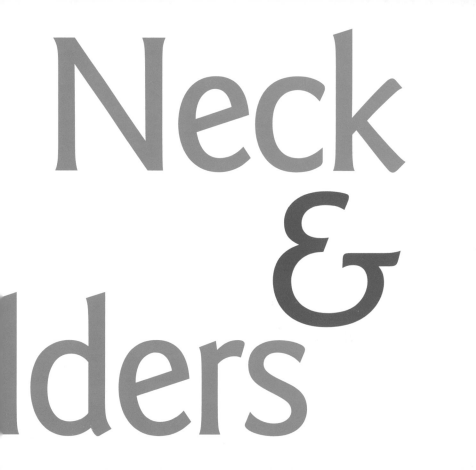

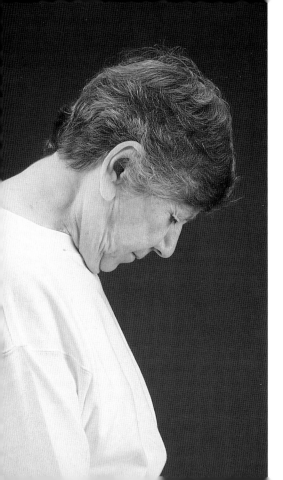

Neck

a simple stretch for upper body and breathing motions

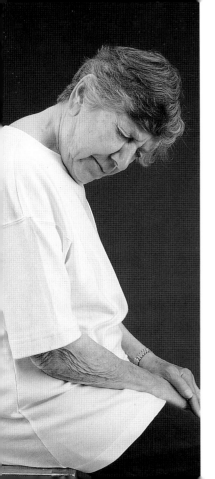

Always be careful with neck stretches, especially if you have had neck problems in the past. Your movements should be slow and deliberate. Never jerk or swing your neck. Consult your doctor if you have any questions.

Sitting or standing, slowly drop your head to your chest. Roll your head to the left so that your left ear is leaning toward your left shoulder. In that position, slowly shake your head "no" two times, first looking up to the ceiling, then looking down to your shoulder. Roll your head down and over to the right side, so that your right ear is leaning toward your right shoulder. In that position, shake your head "no" two times, looking up to the ceiling and down to your shoulder. Repeat the exercise.

a stress-reducing stretch
performed easily any
time of day

Neck &
Shoulders

Sitting or standing with square shoulders, looking straight ahead, shrug your shoulders up toward your ears and hold them there for about 3 seconds. Relax your shoulders down. Repeat the stretch.

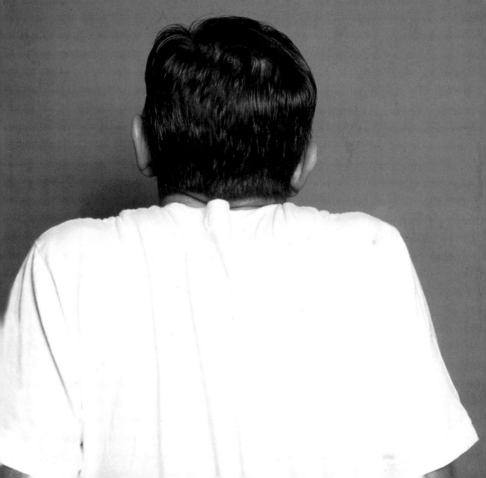

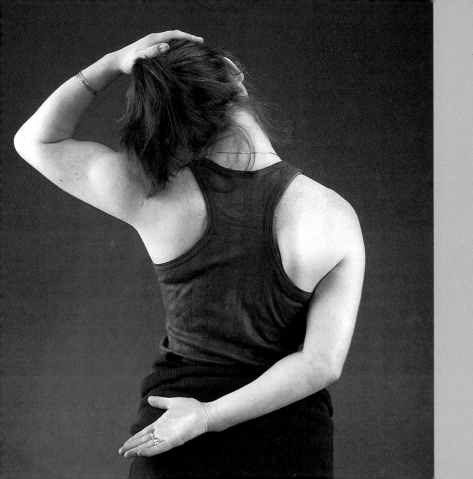

&Neck
Shoulders

a stress-reducing stretch
performed easily any
time of day

Sitting or standing, lean your left ear to your left shoulder. Stretch your right arm down and across behind your back while resting your left hand on or near your right ear. Hold this stretch for at least 15 seconds, relax, and repeat the stretch for another 15 to 30 seconds. Repeat the stretch to the right side. You may also do this stretch by tilting your left ear toward your left shoulder, resting your left hand on or near your right ear, and reaching your right arm out to the side. Hold this stretch for at least 15 seconds, relax, and repeat the stretch for another 15 to 30 seconds. Repeat the stretch to the right side.

Back

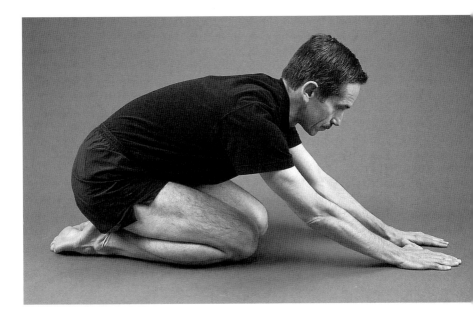

& Shoulders

increased flexibility in this area reduces tension in the rest of the body

Kneeling down with your butt resting on your heels and your arms stretched out in front of you, lean your upper body toward the floor. Once your hands have touched the ground in front of you, reach your arms as far forward as they will go along the ground while keeping your butt resting on your heels. Press your arms and shoulders toward the floor for at least 15 seconds. Sit up and relax. Repeat the stretch for another 15 to 30 seconds.

Chest

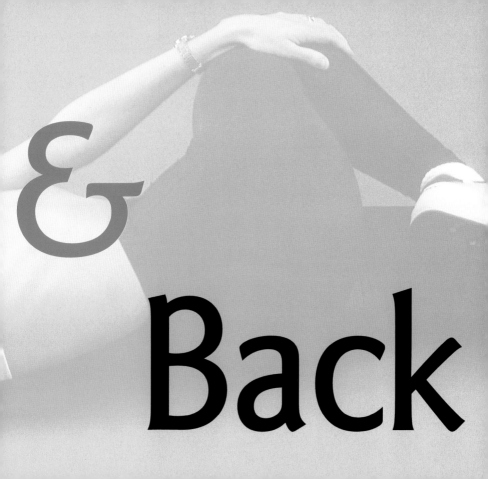

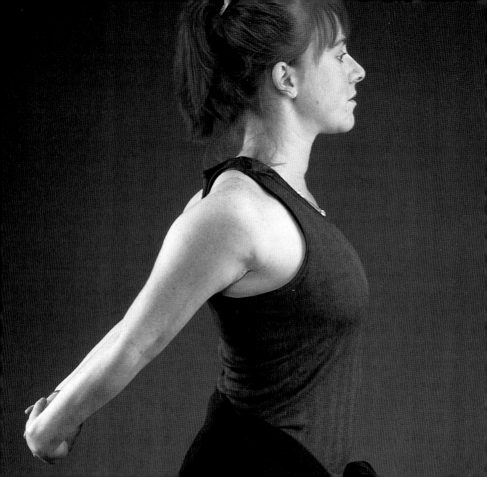

Chest

*an important stretch
for improved breathing
and posture*

Sitting or standing, bring your arms
behind your back and interlace your
fingers with your palms facing inward.
Straighten your arms and lift them up until
you feel a stretch in your arms, shoulders,
and chest. Hold the stretch for at least 15
seconds. Relax your arms, then repeat the
stretch for another 15 to 30 seconds.

Back

*improved flexibility in the
back is paramount to
healthy total body movement*

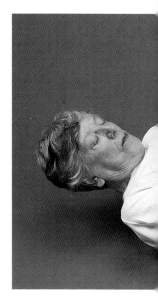

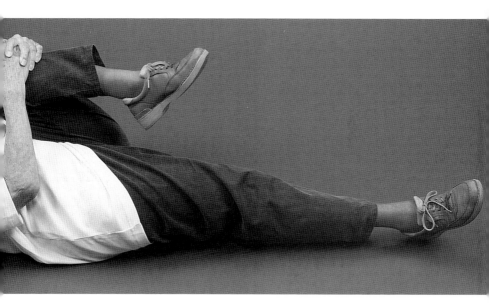

Lie flat on your back and pull your right knee into your chest with your hands. Lift your head and try to touch your knee with your forehead. Hold the stretch for at least 15 seconds, then switch legs and repeat the exercise with your left leg. Repeat the exercise on both sides.

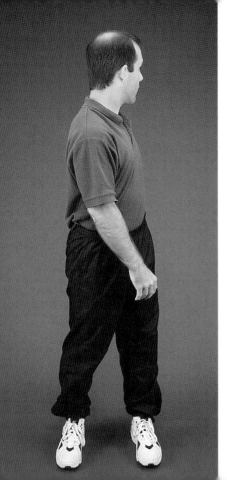

*improved flexibility in the
back is paramount to
healthy total body movement*

Back

Standing with feet hip-distance
apart and your lower body facing
forward, twist your upper body so
that you are looking behind you.
Reach farther by twisting your arms
around your waist in the direction
you are twisting. Hold the stretch
for at least 15 seconds, then twist
to the other side and hold for
at least 15 seconds. Repeat the
exercise on both sides.

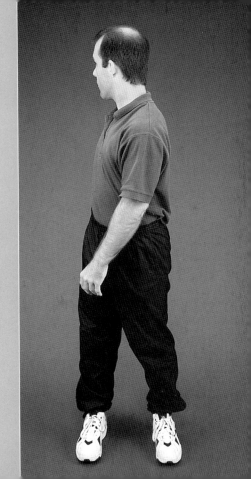

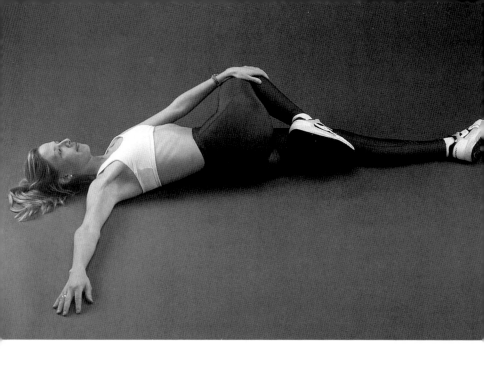

Lower Back

Lie on your back, facing the ceiling, with both arms out to the side. Stretch your left leg out straight and bend your right leg at the knee, keeping your right foot flat on the floor. Roll your right leg over your straight left leg, keeping your right knee bent at about a 45-degree angle to your trunk. Keep your right arm and shoulder flat on the floor as you hold the outside of your right knee with your left hand. Hold the stretch for at least 15 seconds. Come out of the stretch slowly. Straighten out your right leg, bend your left knee, and repeat the stretch to the right side.

a stretch to provide a flexible base for the rest of the body

Abd
&
Groin

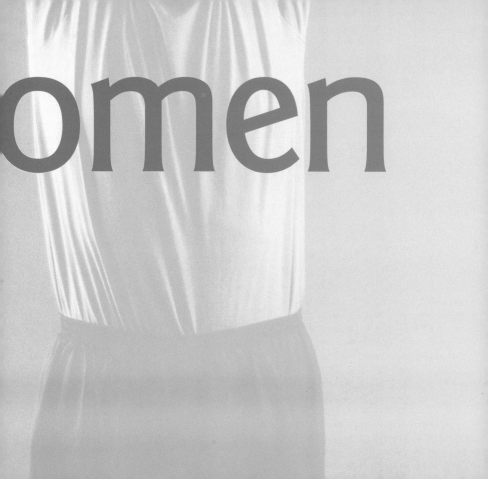

*a flexible abdominal area
is important in the maintenance
of lower back health*

Abdomen

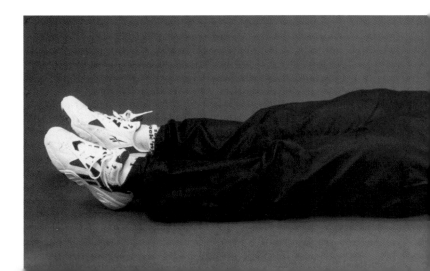

Lie on your back, extend your arms above your head, and straighten your legs. Pointing your toes and pushing your lower back into the floor, stretch your arms and legs in opposite directions for 5 seconds. Relax. Repeat the stretch for another 5 seconds.

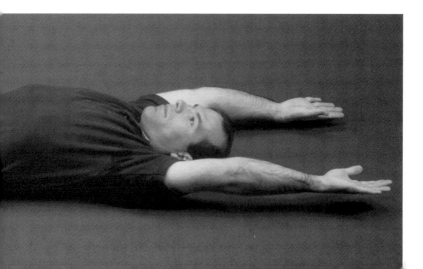

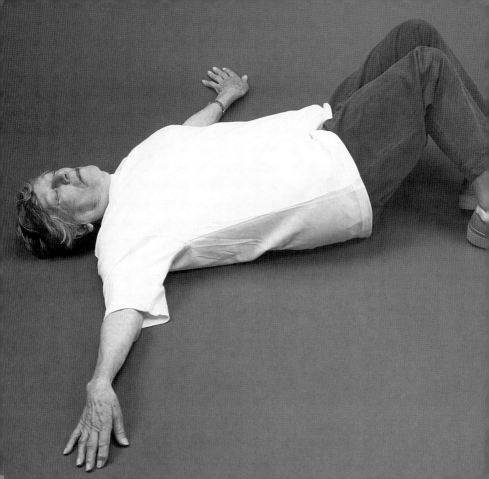

Obliques

important for maintaining efficient breathing and trunk rotation

Lie on your back, facing the ceiling, with both arms out to the side, both knees up, and feet flat on the floor. Roll your legs to the left, knees still bent at about a 45-degree angle to your trunk. Keep both shoulders on the floor as you hold the stretch for at least 15 seconds. Slowly roll your legs to the right, keeping your knees together, and repeat the stretch to the right side.

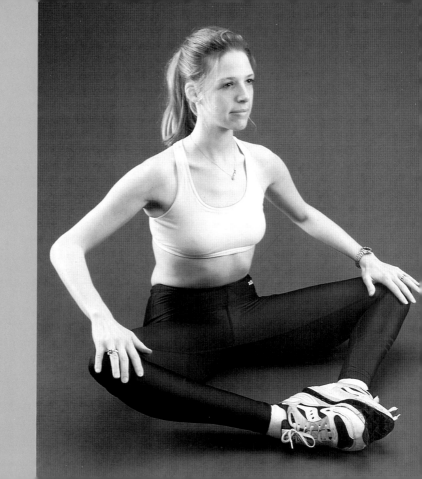

Groin

a valuable stretch for healthy
movement and function
of hips and legs

Sitting up straight, bend your knees
out and bring the soles of your feet
together in front of you. Rest your
hands on top of the inside of your
knees and gently press your knees
down toward the floor. Hold this
stretch for at least 15 seconds. Relax
your legs, then repeat the stretch for
another 15 to 30 seconds.

an important stretch
for overall lower
body flexibility

Hip Flexor

Bending down with knees parallel to one another, extend your right leg straight out behind you. Keep your left leg bent in front of you, your knee directly above your ankle, your calf perpendicular to the floor, and your hands on the floor beneath your shoulders. _Never stretch with your knee in front of your ankle._ Without shifting your position, gently push your hips toward the floor. Hold the stretch for at least 15 seconds, then switch legs. Repeat the stretch on both sides.

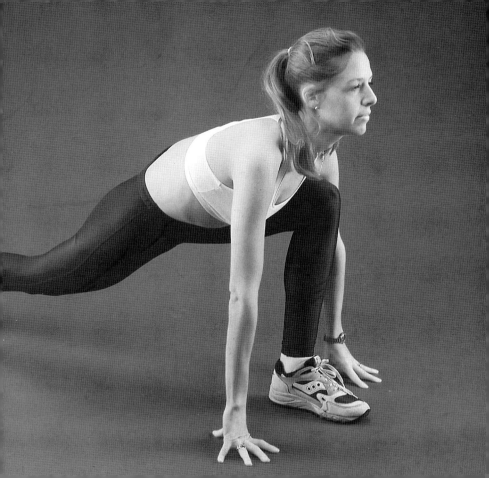

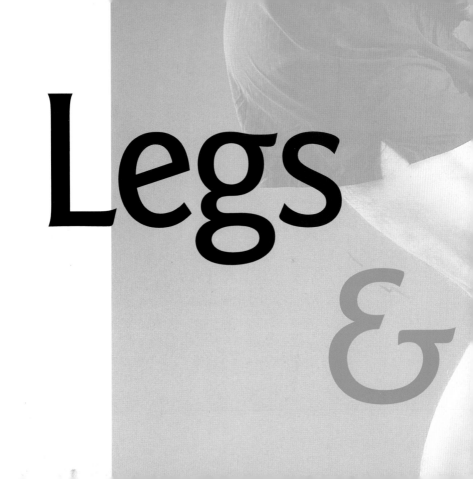

Legs &

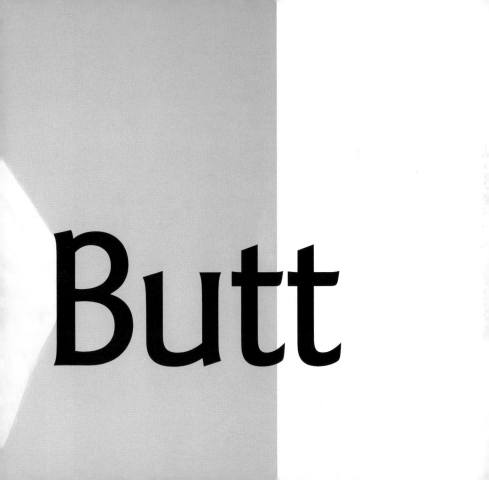

Butt

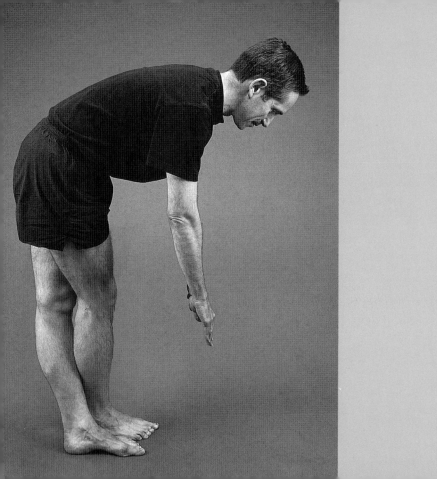

a very important stretch for
effective walking and running

Hamstrings

Standing, cross your right foot over your left. Keeping your knees slightly bent, bend down from your waist and try to touch your toes with your hands. Hold the stretch for 10 seconds. Roll up slowly, cross your left foot over your right, and repeat the stretch.

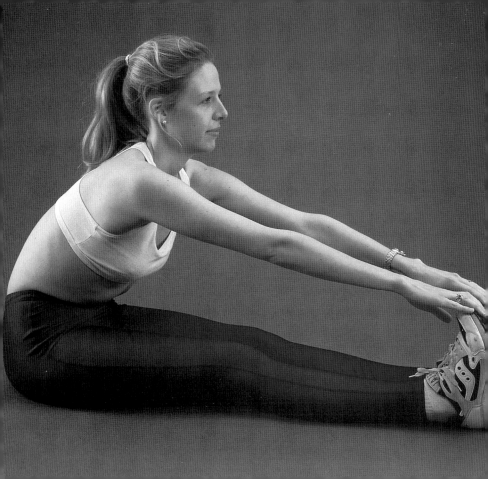

a very important stretch for
effective walking and running

Hamstrings

Sitting up straight with your legs stretched out in front of you and your feet flexed, reach your arms out and try to touch your toes with your hands. Be careful not to reach too far; stretch only as far as is comfortable. Hold the stretch for 15 to 30 seconds. Sit up and relax, then go into the stretch again for another 15 to 30 seconds.

&Hamstrings
&Butt

*promotes increased ease
of motion between upper
and lower body*

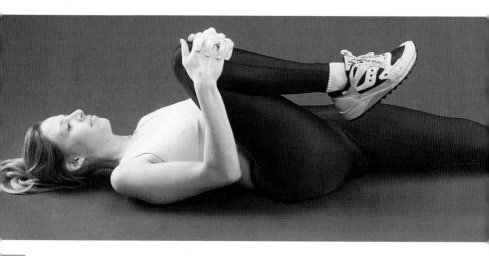

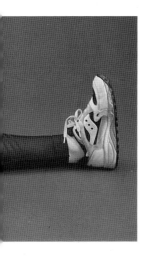

Lie on your back with your left leg stretched out straight and your right leg bent at the knee, right foot flat on the floor. Grab your bent leg just below the knee and gently pull the bent right leg as one unit into your chest. Hold the stretch for at least 15 seconds, and repeat it on your left leg. Repeat the stretch on both sides.

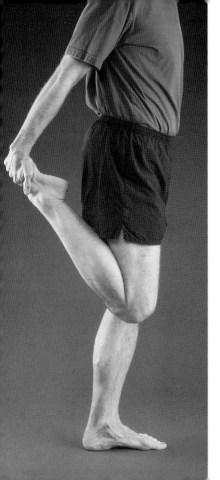

Quad

inactive while sitting, these muscles must be lengthened often for efficient movement of legs

Standing and holding onto a wall or
a chair if you need it for balance, bend
your right knee and lift your right foot
behind you, holding onto the ankle
with your right hand. Gently pull your

iceps

heel toward your butt, keeping your
knees close together and your back
straight. Hold the stretch for at least
15 seconds, then repeat it on your left
leg. Repeat the stretch on both sides.

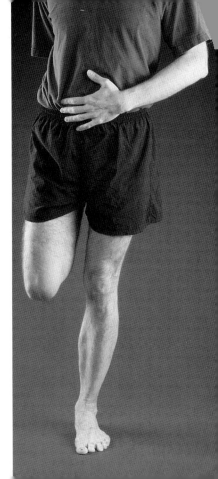

Standing about 3 feet from a wall, place your left foot on the ground in front of you about 5 inches from the wall. Keep your right leg straight behind you. Lean against the wall with your forearms, your head against your hands on the wall. Gently move your hips forward toward the wall, keeping your back flat and your right heel on the ground. Hold the stretch for at least 15 seconds, then switch legs and repeat it on your left leg. Repeat the stretch on both legs. To stretch the Achilles tendon, follow the instructions for the calf stretch, but bend the knee of the back leg slightly during the stretch instead of keeping it straight, so that your heel comes up an inch or 2 from the floor. Hold for at least 15 seconds, then switch legs. Repeat on both legs.

Calves & Achilles Tendon

a simple stretch to relieve tightness in a common problem area and to maintain healthy and comfortable movement of legs

A Final Word

No matter what your fitness level, stretching is one of the most valuable habits you can add to your daily routine. It will enhance your performance and prevent injuries, and it can be a springboard to many other activities. If you've enjoyed the basic techniques in this book, you may be interested in trying a more intense low-impact activity like yoga or tai chi. Look for listings in your local newspaper. If you would like to learn more about stretching as preparation for a specific sport in which you are involved, contact your doctor or physical therapist.